Reflexology:
How to Relieve Stress and Reduce Pain through Reflexology Techniques

Jen Solis

Contents

Introduction

I want to thank you and commend you for taking time to read the book, "Reflexology: How to Relieve Stress and Reduce Pain through Reflexology Techniques.". This book contains everything that you need to know so that you can perform reflexology not only on yourself but on others as well.

In this book, you are going to learn:

- What reflexology is and how it can help reduce the pain, stress and anxiety in your life as well as how it can help to heal your body.
- How to perform hand, foot, and face reflexology, ensuring that you and those you perform it on are receiving the most benefits.
- How relaxation techniques can help to speed up the healing process.
- How reflexology, can help to improve your overall health.
- And more.

When you finish reading this book, you are going to have all of the information that you need so that you can start performing reflexology on yourself as well as on those that you love the most, reducing the stress, anxiety, and pain while improving overall health as well.

Thanks again for taking time to read this book, I hope you enjoy it!

Chapter 1 - Reflexology: Often Misunderstood

So many people completely misunderstand what reflexology is and a simple Google search will prove that this statement is correct. Most people are confused and believe that reflexology is nothing more than a technique that is used in spas to massage the feet.

The truth is, reflexology is much more than a simple foot massage. Reflexology is a great treatment for those who prefer to stay dressed while they are receiving their massages because the person performing the reflexology is going to focus on the hands, ears, and feet.

There is evidence of reflexology being used as far back as 4,000 years ago, by the ancient Egyptians, as well as in China. Reflexology is unlike a normal foot massage, but if the person performing the reflexology is not skilled or is just learning the technique, it will simply feel like a very long massage (which no one ever complains about).

Reflexology is a technique that is used to reduce stress as well as pain by applying pressure to different areas of the body. Each of these areas are believed to affect a specific organ when pressure is applied to them.

Some practitioners not only use their own hands to apply this pressure, but also other tools such as rubber balls, rubber bands, and wooden sticks.

When you use reflexology to reduce the stress in your body, you will find that your body is able to relax, which means that it will be able to heal itself. So, while you may be saying, "I don't really need to reduce a lot of stress," doing so will help to heal all the other areas of your body.

This happens because when pressure is applied to specific areas of your body, the nerves in the specific areas that are being massaged will send a signal to your central nervous system. This message will help to calm your central nervous system and will cause your body to adjust the tension levels in that specific area.

This will cause your body to begin to relax, your organs will begin functioning properly, and the blood supply to all of your organs will increase. Reflexology will not only help you to relax, but it will positively affect your respiratory system, immune system, circulatory system, endocrine system and neuropeptide system.

Not only is reflexology going to help you reduce your stress levels and improve your health, but it can also help you to reduce the pain that you are dealing with. There is a theory, called the *neuromatrix* theory of pain, in which it is believed that pain is subjective. This means that it is believed that what you think is pain, may not really be pain but is instead created inside of the brain.

The brain is going to tell you that your body is in pain if you are physically injured; for example, if you stub your toe or cut your finger; but it is also able to create pain within the body in response to emotional issues as well as mental issues.

According to this theory, your mood, your mental state and the stress that you are dealing with can all cause you to experience different types of pain. The theory suggests that by using reflexology, you can reduce the stress in your life and improve your mood, which will reduce the amount of pain that you experience.

There is another theory that is called the vital energy theory. This theory is based on the idea of addressing stress in the human body. It is believed that if you do not release the stress that you deal with on a regular basis, your energy will become congested, which can lead to pain, decreased functioning of the organs and illness. Using reflexology, according to the theory of vital energy, will help to keep the energy flowing and ensure there is no congestion.

There are a few things that you need to know before starting reflexology.

1. Those performing reflexology on clients are not healing the body, reflexology is not healing the body. Instead, you need to understand that it is the body healing the body. When you visit a reflexology practitioner, you will find that they do not call themselves healers, which is quite unlike many other common techniques. They don't even claim that reflexology is going to heal you. They will need to recognize that reflexology is a technique that is used to bring the body back into balance, to clear the blockages and allow it to heal itself.

2. The self consists of not just a physical being but a spiritual being as well. Reflexology addresses the needs of the mind, body, and spirit. A relaxed body can help calm the mind as well as the emotions, it can help bring energy to the body and help the spirit feel whole.

3. You don't have to focus or concentrate in order to reap the benefits of reflexology. Your body is going to respond to touch which will help to enable healing on every level. You do not have to have any special skill or talent in order to benefit from reflexology. You do not have to change your spiritual beliefs and do not have to focus on anything in particular while you are getting massaged. As long as the practitioner is completely centered and focused on the process, your body is going to respond to their touch.

4. You or the practitioner may actually feel the energy starting to move. For example, if the practitioner is working on one specific point of the body, focusing on one specific system, you and the practitioner may actually feel the energy starting to flow through the body as the congestion of energy is released.

Before you begin reflexology you have to know that it is not going to treat any specific disease or illness, but is instead meant to help relieve the stress and pain that you are dealing with so that your body is able to heal itself.

You also need to know that reflexology is not to be used in place of regular medical treatment. If you are going to a reflexologist, you should feel comfortable asking questions, but it is my hope that you will have all of your questions answered in this book, because I would like to teach you how you can perform reflexology on yourself and those you love the most.

If you are going to a reflexologist and they are not open or willing to answer your questions about the services they offer, you can stop the session and walk away. There is no reason to put yourself at risk or receive services that are not going to benefit you.

Before we move on to the next chapter, I want to go over a few issues that reflexology can help with. Most people turn to reflexology when they are suffering from issues such as: back pain, constipation or other digestive issues, menstrual issues, sports injuries, tension headaches, stress and conditions that are related to stress, headaches, insomnia, hormonal issues, and arthritis.

An average session will last between 45 minutes and 60 minutes and it is best if you can schedule your session at the end of the day because it relaxes you so much that you may find yourself quite tired.

Chapter 2 - Reflexology Zones

As I stated in the previous chapter, reflexology is more than just a foot massage, which it is, but to begin this chapter, I want to go over the reflexology zones of the feet.

Most of the zones of the feet are the same, each foot being a reflection of the other, however, there are a few differences which I will note as we work through the zones.

Let's begin with the right foot. On the right foot, there are many different zones, but we will begin with the 10 longitudinal zones. These zones are what reflexology is based on and each zone will represent one area of the body. The 10 longitudinal zones run the length of your foot vertically from top to bottom.

Starting with the big toe, it is important for you to understand that each toe is going to represent a zone and that zone is going to go the full length of the foot but the big toes will each represent ½ of the head as well.

There will be five zones of the head that are represented in each of the big toes as well. The next thing that you need to know is that the 10 zones are numbered one through five, each foot representing a side of your body.

Imagine that your body was cut in half. Zone one on each of your feet begins at your big toe and goes all the way over to the second toe but does not include it. This line goes all the way up your body. When it comes to your arms, zone one will begin at your thumb and end at your index finger, it will run the entire length of your arm.

Zone two begins at your second toe and goes until your third, but does not include the third toe. It also includes the index finger, but not the middle finger. Zone three runs from your third toe to the beginning of your fourth. It will also include the middle finger but not the ring finger.

Each zone will continue just as the others, from one toe to the next, all the way up to the top of the head and from the fingers all the way up the arms.

So what does all of this mean? Basically, it means that by knowing these zones, you can use reflexology to relieve the stress and pain that you are holding on to. For example, if you are dealing with pain on the outer hip, you would know that this is zone five and you need to focus on zone five during your reflexology session.

Next I want to talk about the lateral zones in the foot. The lateral zones are some of the most important zones when it comes to reflexology. The main purpose of

these zones is to help the practitioner be more precise when it comes to locating the issues in the body.

On the side of the foot right below your little toe, you will find a bone. This bone is where the first line will begin and it will go all the way across the foot in a curved line until it ends just below the big toe. Everything above this line is going to represent the head and the neck.

The next section is going to include the balls of the feet. The balls of the feet are darker in color than the middle of the foot or even the soles, and if you were to draw a line from the lower part of the balls on your feet, this would be your diaphragm line. From this line up to the shoulder line will represent the chest. The outer section of the foot or where the foot is curved is going to represent the arms.

From the diaphragm line all the way down to the top of the heel will be the area that represents the abdomen. If you were to draw a line across the top of the heel, it would represent the pelvic area. From the pelvic line down will represent the lower abdomen. The leg is represented by the outside of the foot, right above the pelvic line.

What does all of this mean? It means you can use the zones to treat a specific area of the body. Another great way to use the zones is to pay attention to where you are feeling pain or where your feet are tender during your reflexology session.

If you find that one area of your feet is especially tender, you will be able to look up the area through the zones and you will begin to understand that there is a problem within that area of the body. Many times, people find out that there are underlying problems with specific organs.

There are charts that go much more in depth when it comes to reflexology, but I am not going to go into these right now. These charts can actually pinpoint a specific organ in the body through your feet, hands, or ears.

There are charts for your hands, ears, feet, and face that you can use for reflexology sessions at home.

Chapter 3 - What You Need to Know

In order to start learning how to do reflexology at home, there are a few things that you need to know before you begin. In this chapter, I want to talk to you about what you need to know if you are learning how to do reflexology.

It is important for you to know that anyone can perform reflexology, anyone can read the ear, foot and hand charts and it is something that I believe every person should learn and add to their health routine.
Not only can reflexology be used as part of a normal, healthy routine, but it can also help you to get a fussy baby to sleep or even treat that nasty hangover.

There are three key benefits of reflexology which we will talk about later; it helps to increase relaxation, decrease stress, and helps to improve balance, and there are only a few techniques. It is also very easy to remember what parts of the hands and feet correspond to the different body parts.

The three benefits of reflexology are of course that it is relaxing, which can help you to reduce the stress in your life and release all of the energy into your body. It will also promote internal harmony and balance throughout your body and systems. Reflexology also helps to increase blood circulation throughout the body.

It is important for you to do an entire reflexology treatment each time you take part in a session, meaning you need to do all treatments for hands, feet or ears. This means that you need to do both ears, both hands or both feet when you are doing a reflexology session. It is important for you to avoid doing small bits of reflexology, focusing on specific organs or ailments during your sessions.

Even if you are using reflexology to focus on one area that you need relief in, it is important to do the complete session because there are other areas of the body that are going to help provide you with the relief you are looking for.

If you are performing reflexology on someone else, you need to remember that people that are not healthy or are suffering from disease can be very sensitive to touch which means you will have to adjust the level of pressure you are using.

Frequently ask if they are comfortable with the amount of pressure that you are using and if the person has been in bed for more than 24 hours, you should not use reflexology on them at all as it will cause tremendous pain.

Creams and oils are not generally used when you are performing reflexology, but are instead used more for massage techniques. If you use creams and oils, you will find that they will make the area you are performing reflexology on far too slippery and you will not be able to perform the techniques properly. You can,

however, use oils at the end of the treatment, providing the person with a deep massage to help them relax even more.

Instead of using oils, lotions, or creams, talcum powder is a much better alternative when you are performing reflexology. The reason for this is that the powder will absorb all of the oils and it will make it much easier for you to move your thumbs over the body. You should choose a talcum powder that does have a nice fragrance because it will help to uplift the mood during the session.

When a person is learning how to do reflexology, it is best if they start with the feet because the feet will provide the quickest results and there is more information available for the feet than the hands or ears.

Ear reflexology as well as face reflexology are great for someone who is feeling overly stressed or that is having a hard time sleeping. It is also a wonderful gift to give anyone that is in need of a bit of attention and love.

Although most sessions will last around 45 minutes, it is important that sessions for the very young or anyone who is ill are not longer than 30 minutes.

There are physical responses that some people display when they are in a reflexology session or even after the session is over. Some people will unintentionally pass gas, their muscles can spasm, they may cough or they may burp as well.

On top of these responses, some people may cry because of the increase or decreases in energy that they will experience, they can also experience flu like symptoms and even feel exhausted for up to 24 hours after their session.

These responses are most common when the person is having their first reflexology session and if they are not drinking enough water (suffering from dehydration).

Of course, all of these responses are short lived and you can help to reduce these responses by drinking a lot of water. Most of the time, everything will be back to normal within 24 hours. If you are providing reflexology to others, you can track how their responses lessen with each session.

If you or the person that you are providing reflexology to is suffering from diabetes, you need to make sure they are checking their blood sugar immediately before their session as well as immediately after. The reason for this is because reflexology can cause the blood sugar levels in the body dramatically rise and drop.

When you are performing or receiving reflexology you need to make sure that both the person performing as well as the person receiving is seated or lying in a comfortable position. If the person who is performing the session is not comfortable, they are not going to be able to focus on what they are doing and they will not perform the reflexology as well as they can. You should never bend over while doing reflexology or sit at an awkward angle. You should also make

sure to position yourself correctly, ensuring that you are not putting pressure on your knees.

While you are performing reflexology, you can also perform relaxation techniques or massage techniques in order help the person you are performing it on to relax. You may decide to break up your reflexology, changing between reflexology and relaxation techniques in order to keep things exciting as well as relaxing.

There are a few different techniques that you can learn when you are learning reflexology but there are not so many as to overwhelm you. You can use thumb walking on the feet since the nerves are close to the surface of the foot. The nerves in the hands are much deeper so you will want to use the index finger to apply firm pressure in a deep circular motion. As already stated, different massage techniques will also help with relaxation during the sessions as well.

Chapter 4 - Reflexology on the Face

There are 15 different points on the face that are used with reflexology and each of these points represents a different area of the body or a system in the body. When you stimulate these points on the face with reflexology, you are helping the person to relax while improving the function of their body and organs.

Relaxation is very important when it comes to reflexology because it allows the person to take time away from all of the stresses and pressures of everyday life. Reducing the amount of stress that a person is dealing with is vital if you want to help them allow their body to recover from what is causing them pain, anxiety, or making them sick.

We all know that stress can affect many different parts of the body as well as many different systems of the body. Stress can cause you to gain weight, it can cause respiratory issues, cardiovascular issues, digestive issues, muscular issues, reproductive issues, sexual issues, and even a lowered immune system.

Stress can cause depression; it can make you feel as if life is simply not worth living and it can literally take over our lives. By focusing on relaxation, you as a reflexology practitioner are allowing the person's body you are performing on to relax, which will reduce some of the effects of stress on their body. As time passes and the body is allowed to relax instead of focusing on all of the stresses, it will begin to recover from all of the damage that was caused by the stress.

In order to perform reflexology on the face, you will use the forefinger or the thumb to apply firm but not painful pressure on the face, on each point. You will keep your thumb or finger in place, depending on which you are using, while slowly rotating the finger or thumb, ensuring that the pressure is being applied with a circular motion. You will continue to do this in the same area on the face for anywhere from 15 to 30 seconds, clockwise. Then you will continue to perform reflexology on the rest of the face, but you will apply the pressure in a circular, motion moving your finger or thumb counter clockwise.

To begin performing reflexology you will want to ensure that the person receiving the treatment is sitting comfortably in a chair and that their head as well as their shoulders are supported. If the person receiving the reflexology is sick or simply prefers to lay down while receiving the treatment, that is perfectly fine as well.

Next, you need to focus on where you are positioning yourself. It is best if you can place yourself behind the person who is receiving reflexology when you are performing it because it can cause the person recciving to become very uncomfortable to have someone standing in front of them or looming over the top of them. If the person is lying down, you can stand to the side of them so that you are, again, not looming over the top of them.

You will begin the reflexology by stimulating each area of the face, or 'reflex'. The only time you will stimulate more than one reflex at a time is when there is more than one point on the face that is for the same area of the body or organ.

You will want to use a reflexology chart while you are working, starting with the collar bone (2 points), moving to the chin (one point), under the lips (2 points), the corners of the mouth, (2 points) above the mouth but under the nose (2 points), the tip of the nose (one point), the cheek bones on both sides of the face (2 points), the top of the cheek bones on each side (2 points), the outer corners of the eyes (2 points), the inner corners of the eyes (2 points), the third eye or in between the eyebrows (1 point), the top of the head directly above the eyes on each side (2 points), the center of the head (1 point), the temples (2 points), the lower chin line on both sides (2 points).

Those are all of the points on the face that you will begin stimulating as the reflexology session begins. Once you have stimulated the face, you are ready to start the session.

To begin the session, using the tips of your fingers, tap gently under the eyes, beginning next to the nose and moving your fingers out to the ears. Rub your fingers gently from down the jawline from the top of the eyes all the way down to the chin, then use your index fingers to rub the chin for about 15 seconds.

With the tips of your fingers, and using both hands, begin moving up, away from the chin to the edges of the mouth, then finally finding your fingers on the cheeks, gently rub them in a circular motion for 30 seconds.

Move both of your hands toward the nose, gently going over the nose until your fingers reach the point on the forehead between the eyebrows, then move your fingers along the eyebrows toward the outside of the face.

Once your fingers have reached the edge of the eyebrows, move them upward, toward the hairline. Rub the hairline gently move over the scalp and the entire head. You can continue massaging the head as much as you would like.

Start the treatment over, moving your hands back down the face in the opposite direction until they are back in the starting position. If you massaged clockwise, move your fingers counter-clockwise as you move your hands back down the face.

As you can see, a facial reflexology treatment is very simple to do and can be done in a very short amount of time. Generally, a facial reflexology treatment should take no less than 15 minutes.

After the treatment is done, you will want to provide a large glass of water to the person that is receiving the treatment, advise them to relax for the rest of the day, not take part in anything too strenuous and to drink plenty of water.

If you find that the person you are giving the treatment to has areas on the face that are more sensitive than others, make a note in their chart. This will allow you to check if the same area is sensitive during the next treatment.

Chapter 5 - Hand Reflexology, Treating Yourself

Of course, this book is not about creating a reflexology business and because of that, I want to show you how you can not only treat others but treat yourself as well. One thing that you will find when you receive a reflexology treatment is that the reflexologist will encourage you to do hand treatment at home on yourself.

That is exactly what I want to teach you how to do in this chapter. I want you to not only learn how to perform reflexology on others, but I want you to learn how to treat yourself as well.

It is important for you to know that while foot reflexology is the most popular, hand reflexology is just as effective and is much easier for you to do on yourself. You can also use the techniques that you are going to learn in this chapter can be used on other people and they are very beneficial because the person receiving the treatment does not have to worry about taking their shoes or socks off and they do not have to worry about having their makeup messed up.

As the person performing the reflexology, you do not have to worry about touching other people's feet or their faces, which can be quite oily.

It is important for you to know that hand reflexology and foot reflexology are completely different from one another. I have already talked about how the reflexes in the hands are much deeper than they are in the feet, which means that you will have to be more firm with the hands and you will have to work at them longer than you will with the feet.

If you are performing reflexology on someone, it is best if you sit across from them at a small table so that they are able to relax and so that you are not stretched across the table trying to reach their hands.

If you are performing reflexology on yourself, simply find a position that is comfortable for you. This can be done in your bed before you fall asleep at night or it can be done while you are relaxing on your sofa.

The same rules go for hand reflexology as face and foot reflexology, you will begin with a relaxation exercise, which we will discuss in depth in chapter 8 of this book. When the session is over, you will want to provide the person that is receiving the reflexology a large glass of water, advise them to drink a lot of water throughout the day and to relax as much as possible for the rest of the day. If you are self-administering reflexology, you will need to follow the same guidelines yourself.

As I already stated, the reflexes, or the spots in the hands that you are working to stimulate, are much deeper in the hands than they are in the feet or the face. For

this reason, it is best if you use your thumbs to apply firm pressure to the reflexes in the hand.

It is also important to know that you will not only be performing reflexology on one hand, but you must perform it on both hands if you want to see the best results.

After you have completed your relaxation techniques, you will begin your hand reflexology session.

To ensure you are reaching the reflexes in the hands, you will place your thumb or forefinger on the area and firmly apply pressure. Moving your thumb or forefinger over this area in a circular motion, you will focus on this area for three to five seconds.

Then you will move your thumb or forefinger to the next area and repeat the process. At the end of the session, you will go back over the hand in the opposite direction before moving to the other hand.

The session:

When you begin the session, you will always begin with the right hand. Just as you would with the face, you want to begin by stimulating the hand. You can do this by giving it a firm massage if you desire, ensuring that you go over the entire hand before beginning the session.

Here is an example of one way you can stimulate the hand:

You can start by using a bit of oil and gently rubbing it onto the wrist. Using wide sweeping motions with the thumb and moving very slowly. Continuing with the same sweeping motion you will move the thumbs into the palms. Work your thumbs from the middle of the hand and sweep them toward the outside of the hand, repeating the motion for about 30 seconds.

Now you can turn over the hand and using your thumbs begin to push from the bottom of the knuckles down to the wrist. You want to do this very carefully and very gently. This is one area that you do not want to use a lot of pressure because it can be quite painful.

Moving on to the fingers, you will begin by holding one finger between your thumb and forefinger and twist your way all the way to the tip of the finger, gently rotating the joints as you move up the finger. It is important that you are firm but gentle enough that you are not cracking the knuckles. Remember, this is to help stimulate the hand and relax the person receiving the reflexology, not to cause pain.

Move on to the next finger and so on until you complete every finger on the hand as well as the thumb. After you have completed all of the fingers, you will give the middle of the hand a gentle squeeze before gently patting the oil off of the hand and moving on to the next hand.

After both hands are good and relaxed you can begin to perform the reflexology on the hand, starting with the right hand.

Applying firm pressure to each area, and moving your thumb or forefinger in a clockwise circular motion, focusing on each area for three to five seconds, you will begin by working on the tips of the fingers.

Starting with the right hand, you will begin with the bottom of the thumbnail, applying the reflexology hand technique I described above, and apply firm pressure just under the thumbnail.

When you have finished the thumb, you will move to the index finger, performing the same technique on the bottom, left side of the nail area. The same area will be focused on when it comes to the middle finger, then on the ring finger you will move to the right side of the nail area. On the pinky finger, you will focus on both sides of the nail.

Once you have worked through all of the fingers, working clockwise, you will work through them again using a counter clockwise motion.

Next, you will go back to the thumb, placing the thumb in your hand, and using your own thumb, work in a circular motion down the length of the thumb. Move your thumb over to an area that has not received reflexology, and work your way back up the length of the thumb. You will continue this until every part of the thumb has received reflexology treatment.

Repeat this process for every finger on the hand, ensuring that every area of each finger has received a reflexology treatment. You may hear a bit of cracking or feel a bit of cracking during this time and that is completely fine as well as normal, but you should continually ask the person receiving the treatment if they are comfortable with the amount of pressure you are using.

It is important for you to take your time when you are working on the fingers because they represent all of the areas from the neck up to the top of the head. This includes the brain, face, ears, eyes, skull, and the glands.

Now it is time to move on to the palm of the hand. This area of the hand is going to represent the torso. You will notice that the areas of the palm of your hands are shaded slightly different. The middle will be just a bit lighter than the top and sides of the hand.

The top of the hand, which is a bit darker than the middle of the hand will represent the chest area. The middle, or lighter part of the hand is going to represent the liver and stomach area. The bottom part, or area that is closest to the wrist as well as the side of the hand opposite of the thumb will represent the digestive system.

Your shoulder area is represented by the small area that is just below your pinky finger (on both sides of the hand) so if you or the person receiving the treatment is having shoulder pain, focusing on this area will provide relief.

Once the fingers are completed, you can move on to the palm of the hand. Place the hand on a flat surface with the palm facing up. Then, begin using the reflexology technique for the hand on the padded area just below the bottoms of the fingers. Slowly move over the area in a downward motion, then back up, working sideways as you work up and down the area.

Continue the same process as you work into the center of the palm as well as the outer edge of the hand until you reach just above the wrist bone. Continue over the bottom of the palm, ensuring that every area of the palm has been treated, then place your thumb on the wrist and gently rub it across from left to right, then right to left.

Turn the hand over and place the palm on the surface so that the back of the hand is facing upwards. Use the same technique as you used on the palm of the hand, but being much more gentle, ensuring that you do not cause the person receiving the treatment any pain.

Repeat the entire process on the left hand. After both hands have been completed, give another gentle massage just as you did before the treatment began, follow up with a large glass of water and explain the side effects of the treatment just like you would if you were giving face reflexology.

Explain to the person that they should rest as much as possible for the rest of the day, drink plenty of water and let them know that they may experience flu like symptoms over the next 24 to 48 hours.

When you begin reflexology, you may feel overwhelmed, you may think that it is just not possible for you to learn it, but as you can see, it is quite simple. If you follow the directions you have learned in this chapter you can provide yourself with reflexology treatments as well as others.

In the following chapter I want to talk to you about reflexology and health, followed by foot reflexology and finishing the book up with relaxation techniques that you can use before your reflexology session begins.

Chapter 6 - Reflexology and Health

It seems today that more and more people are becoming more aware of their health. They are becoming more aware of what they are putting into their bodies. They are more focused on providing their bodies with the fuel that it needs from organic foods and hormone-free meats.

The reason for this is that they have lived through the effects of not taking care of their bodies. Of course, reflexology is not going to completely change your health, but it is a great treatment to add into your healthy lifestyle.

One thing that people are finding is that by changing their diet, they are giving their bodies what it needs, but they are not able to reverse a lot of the damage that has been done. They are also finding that they are in a lot of pain because of this damage as well as because of the stress that they are dealing with on a regular basis.

We have to face it, there is never going to come a point when food alone can heal our bodies, but what people are finding is that when they add reflexology to their health regime, they are able to reverse the effects of the unhealthy lifestyle they used to live.

Not only can reflexology help with stress and pain relief, but it can help with weight loss, sinus issues, constipation, hangovers, headaches, sexual issues, shoulder pain, sleeping problems, sore throat, nausea, and even glandular issues.

You may also find that along with your diet changes and reflexology, meditation might be something that you want to add to your regimen. Reflexology and meditation go hand in hand because meditation will help you to relax and focus on what you are doing instead of being distracted by everything around you.

You do not have to sit down, Indian style with your hands on your knees chanting, but instead you can choose to use mindful meditation. Mindful meditation is a great way to reduce the amount of stress that you are dealing with in your life while keeping your focus on what needs to be done right now.

Think about this, you wake up in the morning, turn off the alarm clock and begin thinking about what you have to get done that day. Before you place your feet on the floor, you think about what you have to make for breakfast, what lunches need to be packed, your shower, the chores, the bills, and your work.

Before you brush your teeth, you are thinking about what you need to make for dinner and how much you dread the day you have ahead of you. Now I am not going to tell you that you should not think ahead. It is great for you to have a daily plan and I will tell you that it is best if you write it down each evening so that you know exactly what you have to do the next day.

When you practice mindful meditation, you are only going to think about what you are doing at that moment. For example, if you are in the shower, the only thing that you are thinking about is the shower that you are taking. You are not thinking about what you need to get done after you take a shower, or after that, and so on.

This can help you when you are taking part in a reflexology treatment because even though you do not have to do anything while you are getting a treatment, you will benefit more if you are focused on the treatment while it is happening.

Why? Of course, I am sure that you have figured it out by now, but the reason why this is going to benefit you is because you are not thinking about all of the stressful things that are going on in your life. We all should know that if we are thinking about all of the stressful things that are going on in our lives while we are taking part in a reflexology treatment, we are not going to get the full benefits.

This is because, as reflexology is trying to clear all of the effects of stress, you are just adding more, and it is only going to counteract the effects of the reflexology.

Don't stop when you finish your reflexology treatment, but instead continue mindful meditation throughout your entire day and life. Doing this is going to reduce the amount of stress that you are dealing with each day and you are going to find that you will be able to get more done than you ever imagined.

We live in a world where we are super busy and our next task is always on our mind, but this means that we are not focusing completely on what we are doing at any given moment. This means that we do not complete our tasks or we do not give our tasks the attention they deserve, which means we are not happy with the quality of our work.

This can also lead to procrastination, even more stress, anxiety, and depression. One thing that we know about depression is that it can lead to pain in the body. Of course, reflexology is going to help these issues, but mindful meditation can take the results to a whole new level.

If you take a good look at anxiety, depression, and stress, it is usually caused by fear. By just knowing this, you can see how keeping your mind in the moment is going to help you reduce your stress and anxiety levels. This will also allow all of that congested energy through your body which will not only make you feel more energetic, but it will help to reduce your pain and improve your health as well.

The great thing about reflexology is that it is a noninvasive treatment. You don't have to go to the doctor, you don't have to worry about taking any medications or any side effects of any medications. Not only is reflexology able to help you improve your health, reduce your pain, stress and anxiety, but it can also help with mental disorders such as depression or even ADHD.

Reflexology is a great place to start if you are looking to start making healthy changes in your life, and it is a great way to begin feeling better and to reduce your pain, especially if you are trying to exercise.

While there is no one miracle cure that is going to remove all of your stress, anxiety, or pain, making small changes in your life while taking part in reflexology is going to help you become a happier, healthier, less stressed person.

Chapter 7 - Foot Reflexology

The most common technique that is used when performing foot reflexology is called thumb walking. Thumb walking is a very easy technique and can be performed for long periods of time without causing any pain or stress on the thumb.

In order to use thumb walking to perform foot reflexology, all you have to do is press the thumb into the foot firmly, bend the thumb and straighten it. The thumb will naturally "walk" up the foot.

You need to know which part of your thumb to use and it is important for you to understand that you cannot have long nails and perform this technique. Begin by pressing the palms of your hands together, then turn the thumbs until they are pressed against each other.
Roll the thumbs up until the tips of the nails begin to touch. The part of the thumbs that are still touching are the parts that you will use when using the thumb walking technique.

Learning the technique:

Begin by opening up your left hand so that your palm is facing you. Place the part of your thumb that you discovered above to be used for thumb walking on the bottom part of your left palm.

Bend your thumb, then straighten it, ensuring that you are not forcing the nail into the skin. As you straighten your thumb, you are going to notice that your thumb will move forward just slightly. This is the technique of thumb walking.

Now, I want you to start again and focus on applying a bit of pressure to the area as you walk the thumb up the palm of your hand. You do not want to use the same amount of firm pressure as you would on the hand because remember, the reflexes in the foot are much closer to the surface than they are in the hand, and you do not want to cause any pain in the foot.

After you have practiced the technique and you are happy with your results. Once you are happy with your technique you are ready to start foot reflexology.

Before you begin the foot reflexology, you will begin with relaxation techniques, helping the person you are performing reflexology on to relax. These techniques will be discussed in the next chapter.

The next thing that you should do is to help the foot relax. When you are performing reflexology on the foot, you will want to begin with the right foot, work on the entire foot and then move to the left foot.

Before you begin reflexology on the foot, and after you use relaxation techniques, you will want to help relax the foot.

Begin by placing a bit of oil on the foot and massaging it thoroughly. Move over the entire foot slowly but firmly, allowing all of the muscles of the foot to loosen. Placing both hands around the foot, place the thumbs in the middle of the foot and begin twisting your hands around the foot, working in an upward motion.

Once the foot is relaxed, you will gently pat all of the oil off of the foot, then you can begin the foot reflexology. Begin by placing your thumb at the bottom of the inside of the foot. This area of the foot is called the spine of the foot and runs from the bottom of the heel, up the inside of the foot (the curved side) and all the way up to the tip of the big toe.

Thumb walk all the way up the spine of the foot from the heel to the tip of the big toe, then thumb walk all the way back down to the bottom of the heel, taking your time as you go.

After you have thumb walked up and down the spine of the foot, you are going to focus on the toes. Beginning with the big toe, you are going to begin by holding the toe at the base firmly and rotating your fingers around the toe in a circular motion while stretching the toe from the base.

Continue this all the way up to the top of the toe before moving on to the next toe and working though all five.

Working on the toes will help relieve any issues from the neck up. Just as the fingers represent the area from the neck up, so too do the toes, so this will help with headaches, bone pain, gland issues, and any other issue that you are dealing with from the neck up.

Next, you will want to apply pressure in a clockwise circular motion to the tip of each toe for about 15 seconds, repeated by applying pressure in a counter-clockwise motion to the tip of each toe for another 15 seconds.

Once you have applied pressure to the tips of the toes, you will move your thumb to the bottom of the toes and thumb walk firmly up the toes, covering every area of the toes, beginning with the big toe and finishing with the pinky toe.

The chest area is represented by the ball of the foot and you are going to thumb walk this entire area, ensuring that you take your time and do not leave any area out.

Now you will move to the top of the foot and thumb walk from the base of the toes all the way up to the ankle ensuring that you cover every area of the top of the foot.

This will give the bottom of the foot a bit of a break from all of the stimulation, which is important if you are working with someone that has very sensitive feet.

After you have thumb walked the top of the foot you will move back to the bottom of the foot.

The stomach area is represented by the thinnest part of the foot and it is the next section that you will begin working on. Begin by thumb walking, side to side in the area that is between the ball of the foot and the thinnest part of the foot.

Once this is done, thumb walk back in the opposite direction over the same area.

This area is very important and you can go over it a few times if the person is dealing with stomach or liver issues.
As I stated, the stomach is represented by the smallest part of the foot and this area of the foot also represents the intestines. Thumb walk across the foot on the smallest section then repeat going in the opposite direction.

The next area, down to the bottom of the heel represents the pelvic area and you will again thumb walk across the area and then back in the opposite direction. Finish with a gentle massage and move on to the left foot, repeating the entire process.

After the treatment is complete you will provide the person receiving the reflexology with a large glass of water, advise them to drink a lot of water for the next 24 hours, explain that they should relax as much as possible over the next 24 hours and that they may experience some flu like symptoms.

Chapter 8 - Relaxation Techniques

As I have mentioned when discussing each of the reflexology techniques, it is important for you to use relaxation techniques before you begin the reflexology treatments. In this chapter, I want to give you a few relaxation techniques that you can use before starting your treatments.

1. Change the environment in order to help you or the person receiving reflexology relax. Play relaxing music quietly in the background, light some candles and dim the lights. Make sure the room is free from clutter and is clean. Hang one or two calming pictures. Having an environment that is completely free of reminders of the stresses that are faced on a day-to-day basis will help the person receiving the reflexology to relax.

2. Lead the person that is receiving reflexology in a few moments of guided meditation or take part in guided meditation if you are performing reflexology on yourself. Spending just 10 to 15 minutes meditating is a great way to help you or those you are performing reflexology on to relax.

3. Deep breathing exercises are a great way for you as well as those that you are performing reflexology on to relax. It's great for relieving stress and good for the health as well. All that you need to do is sit in a quiet area where you will not be disturbed. Make sure that you are in a comfortable

position and begin by taking a deep breath in through your nose. Count to ten as you inhale, hold the breath for three counts and then exhale through your mouth. As you are inhaling you want to focus on how inhaling affects your body. Do not allow your shoulders to raise as you inhale, but instead force your stomach to expand. This is the proper way to breathe and it will ensure that you become more aware of how you are breathing. It will also provide your body with the oxygen it needs.

It is important for the person receiving reflexology to relax before the treatment begins not only because it will make the reflexology more effective, but it will also lower the heart rate, drop as well as stabilize the blood pressure, allow the muscles to begin to relax, and it will allow the body to begin to heal itself. Reflexology will help the body relax the rest of the way, but taking part in relaxation techniques before a session will help to speed up the healing process. This means that the person receiving the reflexology will have their pain reduced, their stress and their anxiety reduced much more quickly than if they did not take part in the relaxation techniques.

There are so many more relaxation techniques that you can use and of course, these are just a few of the easiest but I wanted to go over a few before I finished up the book to show you just how easy it is.

Conclusion

Thank you again for taking time to read this book!

I hope this book was able to help you to begin practicing reflexology so that you can reduce the stress, pain and anxiety in your life as well as the life of others.

The next step is to keep practicing your technique, perfecting it and sharing reflexology with those you love.

If you have enjoyed this book, please be sure to leave a review and a comment to let us know how we are doing so we can continue to bring you quality ebooks.

Thank you and good luck!

Reiki:
The Reiki Healing Guide for Increasing Your Energy, Health and Well-being

Jen Solis

Table of Contents

Introduction – The Basics of Reiki

I want to thank you and commend you for taking time to read the book, *"Reiki:*

The Reiki Healing Guide for Increasing Your Energy, Health and Well-being".

Reiki was originally discovered in Japan during the 1920's by Makao Usui during a mountain meditation retreat. This original form of Reiki is often referred to as Usui Reiki in his honor. The term comes from the kanji of *Rei* and *Ki (Qi)* which translates to 'a guiding of life force energy'. This energy shouldn't be confused with the physical body, as life force energy is more about consciousness and about awareness.

We're often aware that we feel unbalanced in some way but cannot put our finger on why. Pain, for example, is a physical manifestation of energy imbalance. Illness, too, can be a side effect of this, as it compromises your immune system.

Reiki healing is something that can be practiced safely every day, and if you don't feel well, then Reiki can help you recover and feel better faster. *The Reiki Healing Guide* can help you achieve better physical and mental well-being through the techniques we're about to show you.

The great thing about Reiki is that even when you focus on healing one part of your life your efforts will affect all parts of your life and help them naturally return to optimum balance. Once you're familiar with the process of balance, you can also give energy to others using attunement techniques which manipulate the energy field and allow you to interact with the energy directly.

There are many Eastern techniques that rely on Qi energy, so why choose Reiki?

You'll find out all that and more here.

Thanks again for taking time to read this book, I hope you enjoy it!

i

Jen Solis

Chapter 1 – Applied Reiki

The wonderful thing about Reiki in comparison to other Qi arts is that it requires little experience and has no hard rules to follow. There is no extra energy needed from the healer and often the practice is nothing more than creating a guide for the energy to follow on its own. Reiki is what you make of it, and the balance of what you put in and get out can be especially noticeable. Reiki healing can be used to heal yourself or others, and while some people may notice energy changes or light and color changes it's okay to simply feel nothing more than extra positivity in your life when practicing. Since we each experience Qi manipulation differently, some people will only experience it subconsciously through vivid dreams or a more peaceful existence.

Once you've become more familiar with Qi and manipulation, you'll be able to feel it just through a simple touch flowing through the world around you. It's especially important to remain relaxed when practicing Reiki, as your intent should be simply directing the flow of energy rather than influencing it with positive or negative emotion.

Healing with Reiki

Much of Reiki is linked to intention. Having an intent solely to manipulate the energy and not influence it allows it to go where it is needed. The intention of healing with Reiki is as simple as laying hands and asking the energy to flow where it is needed. This can apply to yourself or with another person. By choosing to ask the energy first, it helps to create a respectful boundary, especially if the energy belongs to another. This also creates a reverence for the energy as being part of a force far beyond that residing in the body alone. It isn't important to have a particular ceremony, words, or pose to do this, but many feel that a simple bowed head and namaste position helps to center the body and focus the mind before beginning.

As well as intent, you'll also need to understand surrender. This can be a great struggle for beginners, as giving up control to a higher power is something that many struggle against. These people will often find themselves trying to force the energy down a certain path rather than letting it flow and becoming frustrated that it isn't working. Simply being able to feel the energy flowing through your body without any form of manipulation helps you trust that the energy knows where it is going without being pushed, as long as you guide it. Think of Qi energy as a willful toddler, you want to guide it along the path so it doesn't fall but you don't want to push it, or it will push back.

When healing with Reiki you'll need both intent and surrender to be successful. You'll need to start healing yourself before you can manipulate the energy of others. It's important to be comfortable and confident in your abilities or this lack of confidence can be passed on during such an interaction. During healing you may feel heat, cold, tingling, or even a vibration from deep within. These feelings show the focus of energy in the body, or even just the flow of its existence.

Hold your hands in the namaste position in front of your heart. Close your eyes and take several deep breaths and become aware of your body. Now focus on your hands and bring them a few millimeters apart. Imagine a ball of white light between your hands and energy flowing back and forth between them. Focus on the space between your hands. What can you feel? Continue to breathe and focus.

Qi Energy

This simple exercise should have helped to give you an introduction to how Qi energy feels. Qi energy, pronounced *chee*, is the simplest form of energy in nature. It is universal and includes all forms of energy manifestation. In classical Chinese texts, life is simply a focused amount of Qi gathered together in harmony. Since Qi is constantly fluctuating and transforming it cannot be destroyed or created, only manipulated.

Qi has two forms, identified as yin and yang. These are two halves or faces of the same thing and both are equally Qi. You may recognize the term from the black and white symbol for it. Yin refers to material forms of Qi that are solid, such as your body and the earth under your feet. It is passive and quiet. Yang is more spiritual and refers to feelings, emotions, and is more tempestuous or active. Every aspect in the universe has both yin and yang to it, and these two elements are constantly changing to remain balanced.

Because of this constant change, our bodies are at constant risk of disharmony if we do not respond. To maintain health and optimum well-being, you need to keep the yin and yang of Qi energy in harmony. Disharmony can be caused by deficiency or excess of any Qi manifestation. For example, a physical deficiency of good food or clean air or an excess of fear or chemical toxins. Qi is often transferred to the body in our food so a good diet is also part of this balance.

Avoiding disharmony in Qi is not so easy with our busy modern lifestyles. Multitasking, stress, and a constant need to problem solve all contribute to disharmony. Before making any effort to practice Reiki methods or manipulate Qi energy, you need to cultivate focus and being able to quiet the mind. Meditation techniques are an ideal method for this and the process of Reiki is often likened to a deep meditative trance. Without even realizing it, you already have an intrinsic ability to sense Qi energy.

Think about time spent with someone you didn't enjoy. Feelings of being awkward, tense, and of a jerky passage of time probably accompany this person. When you think of how you felt around them, you didn't feel comfortable or at ease, perhaps they simply "rubbed you the wrong way" just by existing. Much of this has to do with their energy. Subconsciously your Qi reacted to their Qi.

Our energy expands beyond our physical body, often referred to as an aura or energy shield. This outer energy allows us to block or interact with other people. By forcibly causing interaction with the other person's Qi, you were able to feel the disharmony of energy. By now you should be more familiar with the way Qi feels and how you respond to it. Take your consciousness into yourself; are there any parts of your body where you can feel a similar disharmony? These can be emotional areas, physical pain, or even just an overall imbalance if you're not quite comfortable zeroing in.
Spend some time focusing on your body as a whole and noticing if there are repeated points that feel out of balance then take note of them. Similarly, make note of your energy fluctuations around certain people.

Chapter 2 - Chakras

The term Chakra comes from the Sanskrit meaning 'spinning vortex'. There are seven of these points within the body where Qi energy resides, balances, and is either given off or taken in as needed. These Chakras spin constantly at different speeds in a clockwise direction. These points can release excess Qi but can also draw in unwanted Qi from negative elements around you. These vortexes transcend all levels of the aura (spiritual, physical, emotional and mental) which means they allow Qi energy to affect every part of our being. A balanced aura is one where this energy spins together in harmony. This means that our aura is complete, and we are protected on all levels by that energy so that it is taken in and released appropriately. When any of the Chakras are out of balance this creates an opening, or disharmony, which can be cumulative over time.

So what does this have to do with Reiki?

Well, most of us live in constant disharmony. Even if it's a minor disharmony, that loss of balance and stress means that our energy cycle has a flaw so we may feel constantly tired or lacking in energy without understanding why. Alternatively, we may feel out of control or wild without feeling the freedom expected. This daily imbalance causes the flow of Qi through the Chakra points to either become misdirected or blocked. When energy cannot flow freely, we become out of sorts, sluggish, and feel unbalanced, seemingly without reason. A blocked Chakra is one where Qi energy cannot flow through the way it should. Reiki works by helping to get the energy flowing again and bring the energy back into aligned harmony. Since all Chakras are connected, simply working on manipulating the energy from one Chakra alone can have a profound effect on the being as a whole.

The Seven

There are seven Chakra points in the body and each has different characteristics and roles within the being. Each Chakra relates to balancing an aspect of our being, be it mental, spiritual, physical, or emotional, and has a corresponding color. There is a lot of information about Chakras available, and much of it goes deeper than needed to understand the principals on which Reiki is based.

The Crown Chakra – 7 – Universal Thought, Knowingness

The Crown Chakra is located at the very top of the head. If you were to place your palm flat on your skull it would be located here at the center. This is thought to be where our energy connects with that of the universe and where the soul enters/exits the body with the life cycle. This Chakra is connected to knowledge, understanding, and wisdom, and is associated with total harmony.

The Third Eye – 6 – Light, Intuition, Clarity, Awareness

If you've ever seen a picture of a face with a third eye in the center of the forehead, then it represented this. Located just above the eyebrows, this invisible eye represents your inner vision and spiritual awareness. This is where our subconscious and inner understanding resides. It is connected with knowledge and, when balanced, allows the person to use their intuition clearly and accurately. It may also be referred to as the brow Chakra.

The Throat – 5 – Self Expression, Truth, Creativity, Sound

This Chakra is all about communication. It helps us to feel happy by expressing ourselves correctly when in balance. Freedom of communication is an important part of being understood and feeling included. It helps us connect with others around us but also aids in our connection to the universe and higher consciousness. This Chakra helps facilitate communication between the inner soul and our consciousness as well. While it should seem obvious why it's connected with sound, the connection is also because of the vibration in the vocal chords. The universe vibrates at a certain frequency, and with skill, we can raise or lower our own vibration to better match it. Many meditations cause the vocal chords to vibrate at certain frequencies which in turn fosters our connection to the universe.

The Heart – 4 – Love, New Beginnings, Compassion, Acceptance

The heart Chakra is the one where people most often find difficulties. Consequently, it's also one of the hardest to unblock because the person has to actually have input. This Chakra is located in the center of the chest and is also part of the connection from the physical to the spiritual. It is where our feelings of love reside, but it can also provide great peace. When unblocked, we can feel unconditional love for ourselves and the world around us. While this might seem idealistic, it's actually more about acceptance than simply love as we would understand it consciously.

The Solar Plexus – 3 – Spirit, Desire, Power, Energy

Often referred to as the power Chakra, the solar plexus is located just below the breast bone in the center of the body. It's connected with enthusiasm and drive but often has links to self-expression and will. This Chakra has a certain amount of autonomy because it is responsible for providing others with energy. When it is in balance we feel encouraged and driven but also guided with an innate knowledge that we are on the right path. There is also a physical connection to metabolic well-being with this Chakra, as it is right above the stomach. When out of balance, we feel sluggish and may gain weight.

The Sacral Chakra – 2 – Manifestation, Health, Creativity, Sexuality

Located in the lower abdomen, it resides just above the sexual organs. This Chakra helps to nurture our sense of self and provides a playful energy that is deeply connected to our emotions. When in balance we feel sensations much more than normal, be they sound or taste etc. This deep sensuality also fosters sexual feelings and can create great fulfillment. As it is also connected to the inner creative spirit. When in balance, we are much more likely to have good ideas and to accept change willingly. This may also be referred to as the Navel Chakra.

The Root Chakra – 1 – Survival, Grounding, Life force, Presence

Located at the base of the spine where your body touches the earth when sitting in a lotus position. The energy here is connected with our life force and sense of perseverance. It helps us strive to survive and stimulates our need to find things that improve our lives. For those suffering from depression, the root Chakra can be a most important place as it is often a block here that can lead to suicidal thoughts. Because of its proximity to the earth, it's understandable why this energy is linked to grounding. This means that your awareness of the world around you is much more astute and you have a clear connection to the physical world. When in balance, we feel secure and involved in the present, which makes us less likely to daydream.

Once you start to practice Reiki, these Chakras will form the basic positions necessary for channeling the body's energy. In fact, just knowing the information on each Chakra can give you clear guidance on where to focus when dealing with an energy problem. We've already noted depression and the root Chakra but there are also physical manifestations of Chakra energy blocks as well as a connection to the endocrine system. The endocrine system is a connection of glands and hormonal organs that help the body grow and develop normally. While energy blocks can cause physiological issues the reverse can be true as well, and physical damage to any area may block the correct flow of energy. Here is a list of how the Chakras correspond to certain organs.

- The Root Chakra – adrenal gland, large intestine, rectum, kidneys

- The Sacral Chakra – sexual organs, ovaries/testicles, urinary system, kidneys
- The Solar Plexus Chakra – liver, stomach, small intestine, gall bladder, spleen, pancreas

- The Heart Chakra – thymus gland, heart, arms/joints

- The Throat Chakra – thyroid gland, lungs, heart

- The Third Eye - pituitary gland, brain, nose, eyes

- The Crown Chakra – pineal gland

Chapter 3 – Clairs and Crystals

These four "clairs" are about your natural intuition. When it comes to healing with Reiki, intuition is very important because it allows you to feel the energy and know where to direct it. Without good intuition, you cannot heal with Reiki and subsequently once you start practicing Reiki you may find that your clairs also begin to develop on their own. These four senses are deeply connected to spiritual awakening and will also lead to working with crystals, but we'll get to that later. For those whose clairs are strongly developed, they may see, hear, and feel others' emotions clearly and without trying. This can be incredibly overwhelming and even scary at first, which is why it's suggested that you work closely with a knowledgeable practitioner rather than going it alone for energy work.

Clairvoyance

When practicing Reiki, clairvoyance allows you to see the energy within everything around you. This can be a metaphorical, intuitive "see", or for others it can actually be a visual phenomenon. If you know anyone who says they can see auras, then this is part of clairvoyance. While not everyone is gifted enough to be able to see auras and energy so clearly, simply having a feel for them is a start and this can often be nurtured into the ability to see. Those who have clairvoyant tendencies often need crystals to feel grounded in the present, and must do extra work on their root Chakra to keep the energy flowing well. People with good clairvoyance often have strong third eye energy and are more likely to have seen ghosts or entities.

8

Clairsentience

Clairsentience is all about feeling, it's the primary sense used in Reiki, especially for beginners. This is often called your "gut feeling" because it comes from the Sacral Chakra's energy. Clairsentience is an innate knowledge or feeling for the boundaries of energy and the strength of any energy you're working with. This intuition often becomes much stronger with use and the practice of Reiki. The problem many practitioners will experience with this sense is that it can be overwhelming until they learn to separate and release feelings that may be coming from someone else. When working with Reiki on another person this may mean you finish feeling "icky" or drained or that you know something is wrong before even touching them.

Clairaudience

This is the most unusual clair to experience from the universe or from other people; but it also connects with the inner voice, something almost everyone has experienced. For someone who is deeply connected to the universal energy, they will be able to hear spirit guides and intuition from their higher self aurally as well as via the "inside voice". At first, many will find any form of clairaudience difficult to deal with as it can be confusing to work out where the sounds are coming from. This is one of the hardest senses to work with when dealing with aural stimulation that comes from outside the self. When dealing with the inner voice, it means that you're able to experience clairsentience with greater surety since you have a vocalization of the feeling; even if it's only internal. Clairaudience is also linked to the Third Eye Chakra because of the strong connection to self.

Claircognizance

It's quite easy to confuse claircognizance and clairsentience. Both are part of the innate feeling of "knowing" whether the information is right or not. The difference between the two is a rather fine line which is why they can be so easily confused. Where clairsentience is feeling that something is right, claircognizance is knowing that it is right. It is about trusting the information you have, which is what makes it so difficult to learn, since we struggle to trust our intuition without the most obvious of signs.

While these clairs may not be skills needed to start working with Reiki energy, they are important in making sure that Reiki work is effective. These are skills that may develop naturally or that may need some work from the practitioner to become formed. It's possible to work with Reiki energy and not have a strong grasp of your clair senses, but you will always have that question about whether or not you are directing the energy right or truly feeling it.

Crystals

Crystal healing is often seen as an entirely different thing than Reiki, and in truth it is. However, crystals can bring something to the Reiki table, especially if you are someone who is struggling to connect with your clair senses. Even experienced practitioners can benefit from crystals, as they help to amplify energy. We've mentioned vibrations already, crystals can help tune in to this vibration and make it stronger so that it is more noticeable. The reason that they work so well to do this is that crystals themselves are of the earth and part of the very vibration you are trying to tune in to. They are a mixture of minerals and basic elements which have their own chemical properties that make them ideally suited to working with similar energies.

Quartz is the most unique of crystals, which is why it is often used in Reiki practice. We've already looked at how important intent is with Reiki, but when used with Quartz it can actually give you an extra set of hands. Quartz has a unique ability to absorb consciousness, which means you can place your intent into the crystal and use it to transmit the energy while your focus is elsewhere.

There are options for using single crystals and crystal grids when working with Reiki.

Single Crystals

As each crystal has its own unique vibration, different crystals can be used for different purposes. Because of this not every type of crystal is suitable for use with Reiki. Ironically your intuition is the best tool for picking which crystal to use as this uses your clairsentience to connect to the energy and your claircognizance to make the decision. Even if you don't feel your senses are strong enough to make that choice, even a hint can give you the necessary push that it is the right decision. Some practitioners will tell you that it isn't you choosing a crystal, but the crystal choosing you instead.

After choosing a crystal it should be appropriately cleansed to remove any unwanted or lingering energy before your next use. There are several simple methods of cleansing including covering in rock salt or sitting it in a bowl of sea salt water. The crystal should remain in contact with the salt for 24 hours to neutralize all vibrations. Other options include placing it in sunlight, moonlight, or under running water, or the option of smudging. Some practitioners also use Reiki intent to cleanse the crystal and this can be applied while you're using your cleansing method.

Once the crystal is clear, hold it between your hands and charge the crystal with your intent and any symbols or particular Chakra energy you wish to invoke. Hold the image of the symbol and your intent in mind and then visualize it entering the crystal with the blessing of the Universal Energy. Continue to do that until you feel the crystal is full or cannot accept any more energy.

These crystals can now be used in person or for distant Reiki.

Crystal Grid

By creating a grid of fourteen charged crystals, you can continuously send Reiki energy to yourself or to another. This is an advanced technique and can act as a power store for you to tap into if you feel like your energy is low. It's an ideal way to practice Reiki if you find yourself too busy to include a session every day or are feeling that you need more than you have time for. This is much more effective than the single crystal method and can also be used to send distant Reiki energy to multiple people at the same time. The process is similar to the single crystal method, only you will need to choose 14 crystals initially. There are 12 crystals placed in the outer grid, one in the center and a master crystal. The center grid crystal should be a cluster, a double terminated crystal, a crystal

pyramid, or ball. The master crystal should be longer and wand-like as this will help with direction of the energy. While you can use a different type of crystal, most practitioners prefer quartz.

The most common arrangement is that of the World Peace Crystal Grid. This is considered to be the most effective grid because it is used by so many people all over the world, meaning it has a much stronger connection to the universal consciousness. This energy boost can make the healing process more effective and stronger. In 1999, matching grids were placed at the North and South poles where the magnetic field of the earth is strongest. The theory behind this is that it taps into the magnetic field of the earth, equating to the aura for the entire planet, which is where it gets strength. The grids were made of solid copper in a Heart Chakra shape. Many practitioners simply arrange their crystals rather than having a specific plate or grid. Generally, the pattern follows one of the Chakra symbols depending on the intent, or a similar pattern like the Star of Life.

Each crystal should be placed with a positive affirmation, and then the master crystal itself should be charged using an affirmation that includes the intent to charge the grid with light, healing, Reiki, and invoking a connection to the universal spirit. The grid should be charged daily for maximum effect.

Chapter 4 – Practicing Reiki

While crystal Reiki is an easy introduction it is not Reiki in its purest form. Those who are comfortable with their clair senses and their ability to feel energy look to progressing on the Reiki scale. There are three levels of practical Reiki, each of which can be achieved through practice and attunement. The first level of Reiki is intended as an introduction which anyone can take. Many places offer this basic attunement to familiarize supplicants with Reiki energy. The intent of level one is to connect with the universal spirit energy and to open their energy channels. It allows practitioners to better feel the energy flowing through the crown of the head and down into the heart and hands.

For most Masters, level one Reiki is simply the connection and the ability to self-Reiki, since you're learning by practicing on yourself. Originally, this level was split into four separate attunements, and depending on your teacher you may still go through this method, however, many masters simply offer it as a single session now.

The most common side effect of a level one attunement is tingling and burning in the palms of the hands. A level one session often includes an introduction into the history of Reiki and the basic hand placements.

The Attunement Procedure

The original Japanese name for this ceremony is Reiju, which translates as Spiritual Blessing. While this originally held religious connotations it's now considered to relate more to a spiritual state of being instead. The attunement clears your meridians to allow Qi energy to flow freely. At level one, the process is quite passive as the practitioner acts as the channel for the energy and as a conduit so you are connected to the universal life force. The purpose of the three levels is to show that you have progressed to a greater spiritual understanding and to reaffirm your connection to your inner self and the universal consciousness.

The four parts of the level one initiation focus on the head, shoulders, occipital and forehead. The first part raises your body's natural vibration level, which increases your capacity for healing and allows more universal light into your body. The second sends the energy through your spinal column at the shoulders to the entire nervous system. This also opens the throat Chakra for better communication. The third occipital part helps to invoke balance so you have clear thinking. The fourth and final part helps to heal and improve the function of your pineal and pituitary glands, which are connected to consciousness and intuition. These glands help with your clair senses and are the reason why so many people find their senses wide open after the initial attunement.

As attunements are usually done as a group and not in individual processes, the procedure may differ based on the number of participants and the master. Generally, it is decided who goes first and the sequence beforehand. The group then enters a guided meditation. A prearranged signal (often three bell tolls) means you will get up and proceed to the attunement room.

Once in the attunement room, you will bow to your Reiki teacher, then bow to the image of Usui Sensei (the first Reiki teacher). When sitting with your eyes closed, you will place your hands in your lap, often in the lotus position. With a steady and calm breath, you should become self-aware. Once you have become centered and aware, your teacher will start to move around you. During this time, you will feel them gently touch or blow on your chakra points. You may be directed to raise or lower your hands. When the initiation is complete you will again hear the signal.

After the procedure is complete you will breathe deep and then rub your palms together as you bring yourself up to consciousness. Stand, then bow to the Usui Sensei and bow to your teacher. Return to the group meditation and sit in quiet contemplation until your guide returns to lead the group out.

Level Two

The second level of Reiki is usually defined as being Reiki practiced on others and an expansion of the energy channels. Level two is usually only a single attunement which emphasizes the heart Chakra. Students will also be given Reiki symbols. These symbols are intended to help create a deeper connection with the universal energy and foster ability to provide distance Reiki. The symbol can be powerful enough to unblock energy blockages across time and distance. Most Reiki masters will insist that students wait for a minimum of 21 days to three months before proceeding to the next level, yet there are others who will offer levels one and two as a combined class.

The Reiki symbols are considered to be holy to many and while they may once have been a privilege to the initiated, they are now widely known. As standalone glyphs they hold no value, they are not like the Chakra diagrams or hand positions in this instance. In fact, studies done have shown that giving level one students the symbols versus level two has differing results. Students with only a level one understanding of Reiki had less effect from using the symbols than those who had more experience. The symbols should be considered as keys or buttons that will work to trigger certain energy responses. The different symbols are essentially different buttons to connect to the universal life force which the student must memorize.

Traditionally there are only three Reiki symbols but many smaller or modern schools have created their own instead. The three symbols are Choku Rei (a power symbol, Sei He Ki (a mental symbol), and Hon Sha Ze Sho Nen (a distance symbol). Like the word Reiki, these symbols are all named for Japanese Kanji but unlike the calligraphy, there are many ways to draw them.

This level is considered to be practitioner – someone who has learned the basics and can provide Reiki for themselves and others but is not yet able to pass the knowledge on.

Level Three/Reiki Master

There is some debate as to whether level three and Reiki master designations are the same thing. As with level one and two, some schools offer them as a combined course. There is a difference in attunements, which is why most believe they should be taught separately so as not to expose new students to instructors who are not yet ready to initiate others.

Reiki Masters are those who have enough knowledge and experience with energy or symbols to be comfortable attuning others. It is, therefore, possible to have reached the same level of attunement but not be considered a master because of an unease with teaching.

These two levels show deep commitment to knowledge of Reiki and it often takes years before people are ready to progress to this stage from level two, if they even desire to. There are many different methods to teach this level which is why it's important to meditate and decide for yourself which path is right for you if you decide to go this far. The level comes with its own symbol, Dai Ko Myo, which means empowerment and represents all-purpose healing. The symbol is, in essence, the combining of the three previous symbols which promotes a higher frequency vibration. The symbol is used by the master during attunement ceremonies for students.

Dai Ko Myo is generally used before and after the three symbols to empower them and to speed their effectiveness. It is also used for crystals in the same way as a first and last during charging for Reiki. The meditation using the symbol is thought to bring healing energy to any situation and helps to purify on a spiritual level. In addition to Dai Ko Myo, there is also the Raku lightning bolt symbol. This is used for transmission for distance healing and attuning students. There are many different versions of this symbol and it is the final step to seal any energy transmission used by Master Reiki practitioners. During the teaching session, the aura from master and student becomes one, so this symbol helps release any karma created during the activity and to release the energies equally so neither feels drained after the experience.

The Master attunement procedure starts with preparing the students by having them sit on the floor. You will first perform an energy scan on yourself, starting at the feet and working up to remove tenseness and allow your body to be open to the procedure. While doing this repeat aloud, "you are safe and secure at all times." This will not only relax you but help to assure your students. You will then perform the attunement ceremony with each student, guiding their energies.

There are several guided meditation options that can be used during the attunement for students. These include visualizing a staircase of crystal with ten steps, climbing the staircase to the top and then visualizing a white door at the top. The student will then open the door and step over the threshold into a beautiful and serene parkland. Have them visualize it thoroughly, including smells and texture. There is a slide in front of them; remind them not to worry and that they are safe and secure. Have them visualize sitting on the slide and then descending into a rainbow colored pool below. Let them imagine themselves floating in the water and relaxing beneath the warm glow of the sun. The warmth of the water is filling them with peace and happiness. Allow them to be filled with the energy, directing it where necessary. Once they have reached peace, you will ring the bell and allow them to come into the attunement room.

This meditation process is also coupled with physical touches and directions given during attunement. Start at the student's back. You will focus on their Crown and shoulders. Place your right hand on their right shoulder, raise your left arm, and allow the energy to focus here while visualizing Dai Ko Myo above their head. Keeping your left arm raised and left hand upwards invoke blessings from the universal spirit, and aid in helping the student become a loving and serving healer. Cup both hands over the student's Crown. With three deep breaths, draw your Hui-Yin (Root Chakra Energy) in and visualize white light entering through your Crown, along your Chakras and back up into your mouth. Blow three deep breaths through your cupped hands into the student's crown. Visualize Dai Ko Myo entering the crown and into the student's heart. Visualize it traveling throughout their body to the tips of their hands and feet then release your Hui Yin. Walk around the student in a counter-clockwise motion, then kneel in front of them, cupping their hands in the prayer pose. Visualize Dai Ko Myo three times, followed by Cho Ku Rei, Hon Sha Ze Sho Nen and then Sei He Ki. While still kneeling, lift their left hand to their heart while still cupping their other hand in yours. Visualize the symbols again three times. Return their hands to the prayer position and place your right hand over their heart, then sandwich their praying hands over their heart between yours. Repeat the symbol visualization. Cross their hands over their chest and cover them with yours. Feel their energy flowing until you feel the process is complete. Stand and walk counter-clockwise to their back. Silently thank Usui Sensei for his assistance and blessing, then draw the Raku symbol on the ground. Disconnect your energy from the student and imagine the symbols sealed into them. Ring the bell and complete the ceremony by bowing to Usui Sensei and each other.

Once all students have completed the attunement, cleanse yourself and change garments. Return to the meditating students and bring them to the present with a guided meditation. The meditation should be short, using only 5 steps to come to the present.

Chapter 5 – Body Scans

Part of the Reiki process is scanning your body for energy issues or holes. Scanning is a process by which you learn to process the feeling of energy and interpret it through your own body and eventually that of others. When practicing Reiki, you should perform sensitizing exercises so your hands are better able to pick up on smaller changes in energy.

Hand Sensitizing Exercise

While standing, hold your arms in front of you like a zombie. Slowly twist as far as you can to the right, then to the left. Repeat ten times. Drop your arms down to your hips and stand like Peter Pan. Place your chin on your chest and then rotate your right ear to your right shoulder. Roll your head back to center and then to the left. Repeat ten times. Keep your hands on your hips and rotate them ten times clockwise and ten times anticlockwise. Lift your arms back up into a zombie pose and then draw them backward over your head and around again in circles ten times. Repeat in reverse. Bring both arms across your chest in a mummy pose. Extend each hand forward in turn, keeping your fists tight. Bring both arms out to your sides, rotate your wrists ten times clockwise and again in reverse.

This process will start the sensitizing by opening up your body's meridians or energy pathways. It's a great way to start your day as well. Once you've opened the meridians, your energy will flow much better and you can start focusing on your hands.

Place your tongue on the top of your mouth. Doing this helps improve the circulation of Qi in your body. Take your thumb and press it into the palm of your hand hold this pose for 5 seconds, focusing on where your thumb touches. Repeat for the other hand. You should already feel a slight tingle once you remove your thumb. Take both hands and place them in prayer pose, then hold them about 12" apart. Tilt your elbows away from your torso. Focus on your hands and breathe in and out slowly. Visualize a flow of energy between them. Now move your hands in and out as if you were playing an accordion, slowly bringing them together. When your hands touch, rub them together as if you were cold.

Your hands should now feel warm or pulsing. This is your Qi flowing and you are now ready to scan the rest of the body. This pulse should remain regular if the energy is flowing correctly.

Scanning Aura

When scanning an aura, you'll be interacting with another energy so it's a good idea to ground yourself. Dr. Judith Orloff has some great techniques for protecting your own energies during this process and it's advised to have some strategy to protect yourself before interacting with energies that are not your own. You can also use this same process on yourself, but you will still need grounding.

Press the tongue to the top of your mouth, you should have already sensitized your hands using the previous exercise and opened your meridians. From a distance of about four yards, walk around the person with your hands outstretched. Concentrate on your hands and slowly move closer until you feel a heat or tingling. The width of the aura may change, so you may see a difference at the waist, feet, back, or head but generally, auras are egg shaped. Move into their aura space a little, continuing to focus on your hands. This inner area is their health aura and you may feel pressure or heat where energy is flowing and an absence where it is blocked. Continue to move closer until your hands are about 5" away from their skin. This is their inner aura. Start on the right side, paying special attention to Chakra points and organs. Most people suffer with energy blocks in the spine even if they have no physical symptoms. Chakra points may feel cooler instead of warm in some people. Move down the body, starting from the head, noting any observations for blocked energy or hot/cold spots. You may also close your eyes to help you focus more on the sensations in your hands.

Return to problem areas where the energy did not feel right. Using your hands, determine how high or low the distortion is then using both hands visualize molding the energy up or down as necessary until it is smooth. Hollows are caused by energy being siphoned off and Qi becoming depleted, it can also be a sign of a severely blocked Chakra or one that is filled with negative energy. Areas where energy protrudes from the body also indicate a blocked Chakra where the energy has become stagnated and built up over time. The block may cause the Chakra to over-activate and continue to try and clear the energy itself while instead it simply becomes congested. Using the same process, use Reiki energy to push away the block and draw the energy back into alignment, do not try and shove it back into the body as this will only block the Chakra further. You may also find that some organs have protrusions on one side and hollows on the other, this can be an indication of disease. Remember that you are not a medical practitioner and should not try and diagnose any disease, but can advise the person to get checked out.

Pendulum Scanning

Unlike using just your hands, the process of using a pendulum can be a second opinion to confirm what you're feeling. A pendulum can be anything, there are people who use items as simple as a paperclip while others prefer crystals for effect. They can be wood, stone, crystal, metal, it really doesn't matter as long as it is suspended and you feel comfortable with the item. Choose something that feels like an extension of yourself. Generally, most people hold their pendulums in their dominant hand, but it should be whichever feels most comfortable. Before each use, your pendulum should be cleansed with the same process as we saw for crystals. While it isn't essential to use this, you still need to use intent when cleansing and visualize impurities and bad energy being washed away. You can program your pendulum to do certain tasks after it's cleansed, some prefer to keep it as a blank slate or to put healing energy into the pendulum.

To use the pendulum to scan, proceed as you would with an aura scan until you are in the inner aura. Ask aloud that the pendulum show you the direction for positive healing energy and note which direction it swings in. Do not try and influence it. Repeat the question for negative flow. Thank the universal energy. Your pendulum is now ready to be used. While the client is laying down, scan their body's energy in the same way you would with your hands, holding the pendulum in one and feeling the person's energy with the other. If the pendulum swings in the direction of correct energy then it is flowing fine, if it swings fast then it is strong energy but may also indicate a build-up or blockage. A small or tight swing may indicate weakened energy flow. An oval shape indicates turmoil or distortion in the energy from any Chakra. A stationary pendulum indicates a total blockage or illness in the area and Reiki should be done with caution.

Pendulum healing is harder to read than simple hands and tends to only be practiced by experienced Reiki practitioners. Barbara Ann Brennan has a great book on using pendulums to heal if you are interested in knowing more about their use.

Conclusion

Thank you again for taking time to read this book!

I hope this book was able to help you to learn more about Reiki and the ways of energy healing.

The next step is to start by working on yourself. You can learn the basic steps of energy work on your own, but when it comes to working with others or proceeding to distance healing it's a good idea to work with an experienced Reiki master.

If you have enjoyed this book, please be sure to leave a review and a comment to let us know how we are doing so we can continue to bring you quality books.

Thank you and good luck!

Preview of: Meditation: How to Relieve Stress by Connecting Your Body, Mind and Soul
Introduction

Thank you for taking the time to read the book, *"Meditation: How to Relieve Stress by Connecting Your Body, Mind and Soul"*.

In this day and age, it's not easy to keep your sanity in check. With all the work you have to do, and everything else you have to handle, sometimes, your mind really suffers. And when that happens, it'll be hard for you to continue with what you're doing.

However, it doesn't mean there's no answer to your problems anymore. With the help of this book, you'd learn various meditation techniques that could take your stress away, and help you get connected to your mind, body, and soul!

When you get in tune with your mind, body, and soul, it will be easier for you to understand what's going on with your life, and in your world. And with that, you can be a better, more productive person—and that's exactly the kind of person you'd like to be!

Keep reading this book now to find out how!

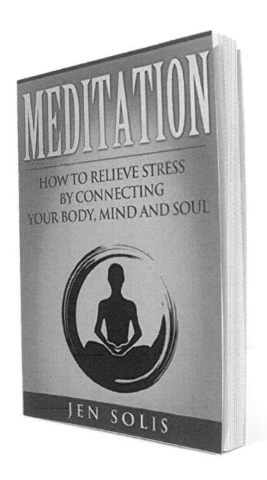

Search for the book on amazon to find it!: "MEDITATION: How to Relieve Stress By Connecting your Body, Mind and Soul"

Check out my book on Mindfulness!

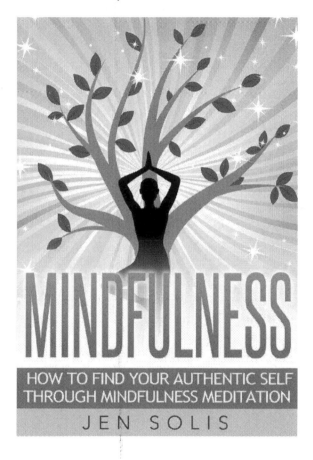

Search for the book on amazon to find it:!: "Mindfulness: How to Find Your Authentic Self through Mindfulness Meditation"

Made in the USA
Coppell, TX
06 June 2022